I0439756

Trigger Point Therapy

Stop Your Muscle & Joint Pain with Tennis Ball Self Massage & Pressure Points

Table of Contents

Copyright

Introduction

This book, *"Trigger Point Therapy: Stop Your Muscle & Joint Pain With Tennis Ball Self Massage & Pressure Points"* is all about how to manage common muscle and joint pains using simple techniques called trigger point massage.

Most people experience muscle and joint pains as a result of activities they engage in, poor body posture, fatigue or strain. Everyday activities such as working in front of a computer all day, construction work, and sports can cause pain. It may also come from simple everyday activities such as carrying groceries, a baby, even a bag. These are recurrent activities that bring about recurrent and chronic pain. Long term pain medications to treat these aches and pains are potentially dangerous for health.

The good news is that something safe and highly effective can be done. It does not even cost much. A simple tennis ball is all you need to roll those pains away.

In this book, you will learn and understand:

- What are trigger points

- What causes muscle pains

- What is trigger point massage

- How to ease pain in different body areas with the use of a tennis ball

Want to know more? Read on and find out.

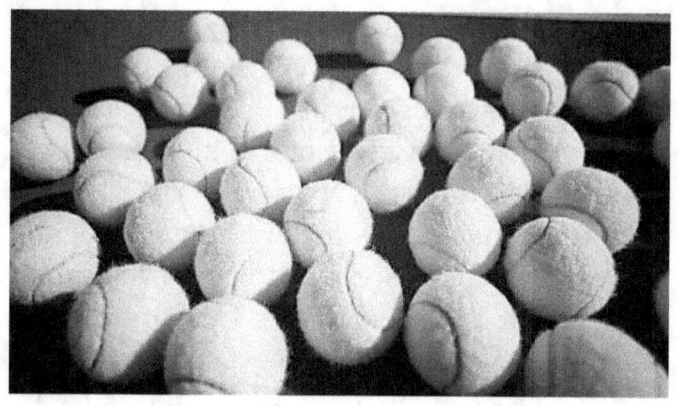

Chapter 1: Brief Glance at Trigger Points

Tight and painful areas in a stretch of muscle are called trigger points. They feel like tight bands or knots within a muscle and are often tender when pressed. Healthy muscles do not have trigger points, are not tender and definitely not painful when pressed. Relaxed healthy muscles are pliable and soft when touched, not dense or hard. These knots are actually constricted areas that appear small and thickened within the muscle fiber. The relaxed muscle areas surrounding the trigger points appear thinner than normal.

Contracted muscle portions can no longer be used. They can no longer contribute to the muscle function because their actions are restricted by the trigger points. The longer these contracted areas are present in the muscle, they produce health problems. They stimulate the release of chemicals that promote pain. They also contribute to a few changes in the structure of the muscles. The affected muscles have to compensate for the limitations imposed by the contracted areas. These changes may or may no longer be reversible. It depends on how long the contractures were present before they were treated.

Untreated trigger points can cause more serious injuries to the affected muscles and adjacent structures. The contracted areas in the muscles can cause the fibers surrounding it to detach from the rest of the muscle. These detached fibers then retract to opposite ends, leaving a hole around the knot.

Symptoms

Pressing on the trigger points elicits the most common symptom- pain. There are also some symptoms that affect other organs aside from the muscles. This includes dizziness, weakness in the knees, sweating, urinary frequency, ringing sensation in the ears and increased tear production in the eyes.

The presence of trigger points may also stimulate adjacent muscles to contract. This will result to loss of coordination and muscle weakness. It also causes the affected muscle groups to become intolerant to activity. That is, they fatigue very easily. Most people think that muscle weakness, easy fatigability, and activity intolerance mean they need to perform muscle strengthening exercises. Engaging in this type of exercise would only lead to worsening of the symptoms. Other muscle groups would be forced to compensate for the decreased function of the affected muscles. This would lead to wider scope of muscle weakness and de-conditioning. Muscle function only improves when the trigger points are adequately treated.

Range of motion becomes limited because of the pain. The amount of restriction depends on what muscle groups are affected, how long the problem is present and the extent of the trigger points. Some muscle groups are more likely to suffer limited range of motion than others. The normal functions are often effectively restored once the trigger points are relieved.

Easily fatigability is due to the ineffective and limited muscle contraction and relaxation. The muscles take longer to return to their relaxed state once muscle activity stops. Also, they cannot fully relax and recover because of the contracted areas.

Also, most people experience tenderness on the opposite side of the trigger point. They think that it is a new and separate problem from the trigger point. In reality, the non-painful side is more-tender. This is because the opposite side is forced to compensate for the restrictions by the affected side. Most of the time, these areas suffered trigger points earlier than the current one. For example, the left side of the upper back feels stiff, tender and painful. After a few days, the right side also feels tender. Most people think that this new tender area is caused by another, totally different, and separate problem. Most often, the right side was the 1st area to suffer trigger points. The body released numbing chemicals over the area, which eliminated the pain but not the trigger points. The currently painful side has not yet reached the numbing stage.

Risk Factors

Studies have found that more women suffer more from trigger point issues than men. Also, teenagers (both males and females) and menopausal women have higher tendencies for this condition. This has led experts to believe that hormonal changes may play a factor in determining the risk for this condition.

Regular exercise significantly decreases the risk for the development of trigger points. People who engage in regular exercise have lower risks. People who overuse their muscles and over do their exercises have higher risks.

How Trigger Points Develop

There is no definite theory yet on how trigger points develop. One widely accepted hypothesis is the presence of an energy crisis. Energy is crucial for all chemical and metabolic processes, and for proper tissue and organ function. Energy requirements of the muscles are provided by a cellular organelle called the sarcoplasmic reticulum. The entire energy process happens in a series of complex pathways. Energy is released by the sarcoplasmic reticulum as ionized calcium. Once released, it acts on the different structures within the muscle fiber, allowing it to contract and relax in a rhythmic, efficient manner.

The function of the sarcoplasmic reticulum is regulated in part by the motor endplate. This is the terminal portion of a neuron that helps regulate motor muscle function. The motor endplate releases ACh or acetylcholine into the junction between the muscle and the neuron (called the neuromuscular junction or NMJ). ACh signals the sarcoplasmic reticulum to start releasing ionized calcium. Normally, once the nerve endings or the motor endplate stops releasing ACh, the sarcoplasmic reticulum also stops releasing calcium. Muscle contraction will cease, causing the muscles to relax. Some conditions lead to increased ACh levels or prolonged action on the sarcoplasimic reticulum. This leads to too much calcium released. There would be prolonged and sustained muscular contraction.

This is often restricted to a small area within the muscle fiber. The presence of contracted muscle fibers leads to higher demand for energy. The sustained contraction also impedes circulation to the muscles. When circulation is cut off, the function of the sarcoplasmic reticulum is compromised. Lack of oxygen and calcium from the blood causes decreased available energy. The muscle remains in the contracted state and a vicious cycle ensues. Sustained contraction demands higher energies but the sarcoplasmic reticulum is unable to provide it. Sustained contractions also put undue strain on the ends of the muscle fiber, causing it to become tender and painful. It also causes adjacent structures to compensate, which causes the "spread" of the problem.

Characteristic of Trigger Point Pain

Pressing trigger points often elicit pain and other symptoms. That is, when pressing knot in the back muscles may trigger pulsing pain over the temples. However, this is not always the case. The absence of pain when pressing on trigger points does not rule it out as a trigger point.

Pain related to trigger points is more often felt elsewhere in the body. It is not commonly felt directly over where the tight spots are. For example, a trigger point is located in the back but the pain is felt on the neck area. This type of pain is called referred pain. Also, in the same example, the pain in the neck may be felt over the head. The neck acts as the satellite trigger point.

The pain follows common "referral patterns", which are pathways that pain from the trigger point follow and end. This makes it easier to locate the trigger point based on the location of the referred pain. About 74% of trigger points are not located directly over where the symptoms are felt. Massaging over the painful area will not result to relief, unless the trigger point itself is massaged.

Pain levels also vary. It depends on the amount of stress that the muscle is subjected to. It is also influenced by precipitating factors. These are factors that trigger the sensation of pain and worsen it.

Pain may be felt as a dull ache, or sharp and intense. Numbness, burning sensation or tingling are indications that the trigger points are encroaching or putting pressure on adjacent nerves.

Active trigger points produce referred pain. Trigger points become active when they are stimulated. The pain is set off by direct blows to the muscle, injuries, inappropriate body mechanics, poor body posture, irritation of the nerve root or from repetitive muscle use. There are also several precipitating factors that can indirectly stimulate the trigger points and produce pain. Active trigger points eventually become latent. The pain ceases without any intervention. When they are latent, trigger points produce weakness in the muscle, with restricted range of motion.

However, pain cessation often leads the sufferer to think that the muscle problem is already solved. Latent trigger points can turn into active ones at any time. The resurgence of pain is often considered as a new problem. However, it is really an old problem that is once again causing pain. Reactivation may come from over-stretching the muscles, chilling or overuse.

It may be surprising for some that by applying only a small amount of simple massage with the thumbs or simple items, pain is effectively relieved.

One researcher wrote that a trigger point can be effectively relieved by just about any type of physical intervention. The simplest and cheapest form of pain relief, and one that is most effective, is by performing self-massage.

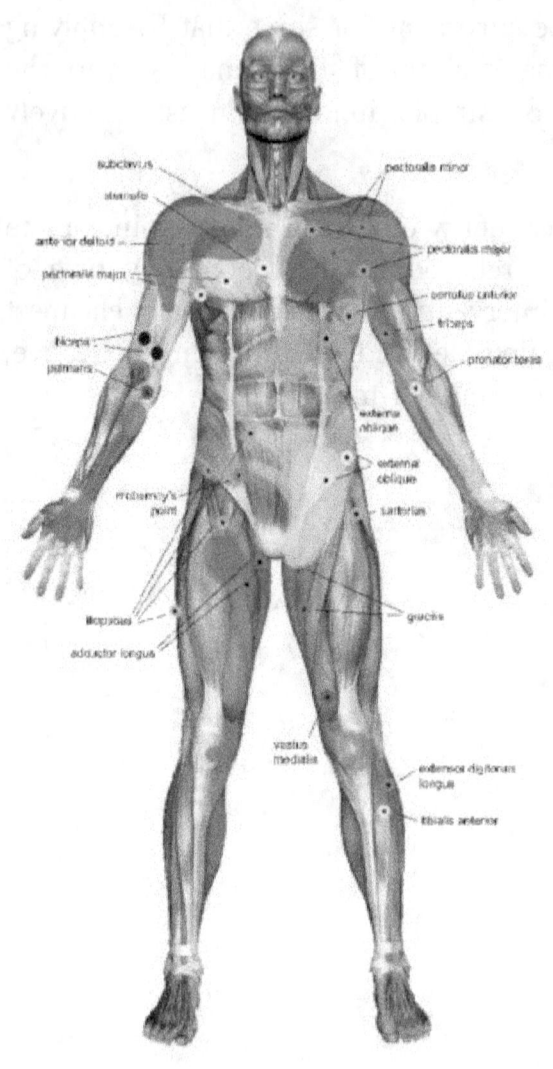

Source: http://www.mastermassagetables.com/blog/

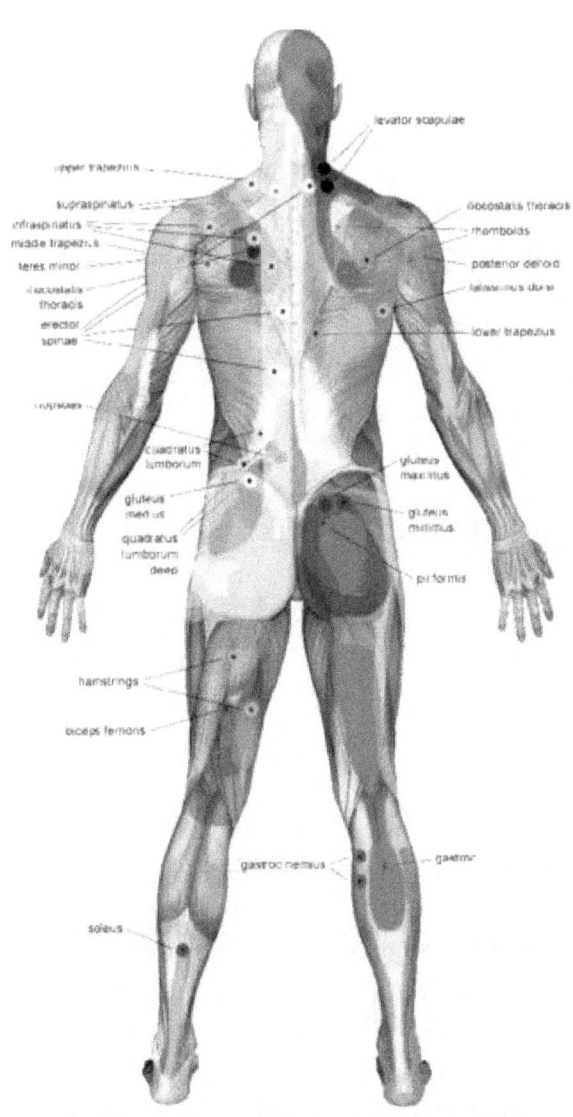

Source: http://www.mastermassagetables.com/blog/

Chapter 2: Trigger Point Massage

This method is designed to target trigger points in order to relieve pain in the affected areas. Like the abovementioned example, headache and neck pain may be relieved by applying the massage method to the trigger point found in the back muscles.

Pain is relieved by cycles of applying and releasing pressure.

Guidelines to Using the Tennis Ball

The tennis ball is a simple, inexpensive but very effective tool that can be used in treating trigger points. Best results are obtained with proper use and execution.

- To find the trigger point, roll the ball over an area (e.g., shoulders, upper back, etc) until knots or pain is felt. Once the trigger point is located, rest the area over the tennis ball or press on the ball for about 2-4 minutes. The pressure from the ball would smooth and release the knotted fascia.

- Pressure should be gentle and sustained. It should be enough to cause a bit of "pain" but not so much as to cause the muscle to feel sore or uncomfortable.

- Trigger points and pain are over the muscle tissues, not the bones. Do not put the tennis ball right over the joints or bones because it would cause bruising and other injuries.

- Sometimes, muscles need to be warmed up first before applying the tennis ball massage. This is especially so with muscles that have been knotted for quite a long while. The direct pressure may cause it to contract even more. Relax them by applying a heating pad or have a hot bath before doing the tennis ball trigger point massage.

- It is very important to listen to how the body reacts throughout the massage. If pain intensifies or other problems surface, stop the massage. For example, when massaging the back, stop if the shoulders, other parts of the back, or the arms start to feel numb or tingly. The pressure may be constricting the nerves in these areas.

Chapter 3: Trigger Point & the Piriformis

The piriformis is one of the muscles found in the hips. It is one of the most common areas where trigger points tend to develop. Trigger points in the piriformis often cause pain over the gluteal and/or pelvic areas. This condition is often referred to as "piriformis syndrome". Women have much higher risks in developing this condition than men, at a 6:1 ratio.

Symptoms of Piriformis Trigger Points

Trigger points in the piriformis muscle causes the entire tissue to enlarge. Adjacent blood vessels and major nerves such as the sciatic are compressed as a result of the muscle enlargement. The pain is most often referred to the sacroiliac region. This is the area where the larger portion of the pelvic bone and the sacrum meet. Pain is also referred to the buttocks and downwards to the back portion of the thighs.

If nerve compression is present, the pain may be felt downwards towards the calf and the sole of the affected foot. The muscles of the buttocks (gluteal muscles) may shrink (atrophy). The leg swells and the foot feels numb and unable to bear weight. These symptoms could impair the ability to walk comfortably. Pain is often worse in the sitting position. Activities that involve weight bearing on the legs also worsen the pain.

If the pudendal nerve is involved, it may cause problems such as impotence in men and painful intercourse in females. Pain is referred to the groin or around the front portion of the anus.

Other symptoms include difficulty crossing the legs while in a sitting position. The foot of the affected limb tends to rotate out of alignment (outwards and sideward) when lying down.

Causes and precipitating factors

Formation of trigger points and pain are related to the following activities:

- Lying or sitting down with most of the body weight on the buttocks

- Sitting with most of the body weight resting on the foot

- Sitting with the knees bent in front

- Sudden muscle overload

- Direct trauma or injury to the muscle

- Twisting towards the side when bending or when lifting heavy objects

- Forceful body rotation while balancing on 1 leg

- Repeated body twisting while throwing something over the back

- Running

- Legs spread during intercourse

- Long periods of driving

- Pronation of the foot

- Long 2nd toe

- Uneven lengths of the legs(one is shorter than the other)

- Chronic PID (pelvic inflammatory disease)

- Joint in the sacroiliac area is out of alignment

- Infectious sacroiliitis

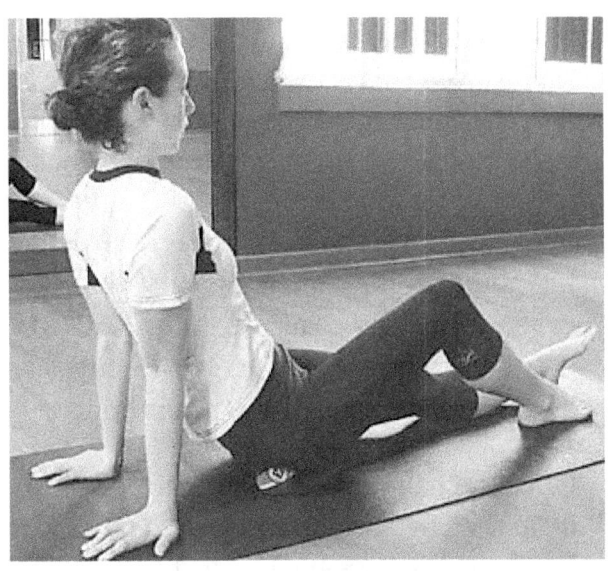

Source: http://fitness4backpain.com/foam-rolling-and-trigger-release-for-your-piriformis/

How to apply Tennis Ball Trigger Point Massage

To apply pressure for trigger point massage on the buttocks, follow these steps:

- Lie on the floor or firm bed, facing upwards. Bend the knees for better posture and stability. It also allows the muscles in the back and buttocks to relax.

- Place the ball over the buttocks and slowly roll to find the trigger points.

- Start with the ball over the edge of the sacral area. This is the triangular bony area between the tail bone and the lumbar spine (lower back).

- Slowly roll the ball outwards, towards the hip joint. Follow an imaginary line that runs from the sacrum until halfway between the lower curve of the buttocks and the top portion of the pelvic bone.

- Once the ball reaches the hip joint, slowly drop the knees outwards towards the side. Keep the knees bent. Most often, the trigger point is located within this area.

Massage the muscles along the spine. These muscles are often involved, depending on how long the trigger points were present and the severity of the condition. To exercise the spinal muscles and improve piriformis trigger points, follow these easy steps:

- Lie face-up on the floor or on a firm bed. Bend the knees. Place a tennis ball underneath the shoulder, one inch from the spine. Hold it in place for 8 to 60 seconds. Slowly roll the ball downwards, holding it in place at each spot. Continue doing this until the ball reaches the top of the pelvic bone. Repeat this on the other side of the spine. Do not place the ball or put any pressure directly on the bones of the spine.

- When the ball is on the lumbar area (lower back), use the hand to roll the ball. Do not lie directly on the ball as this may cause further injuries.

Chapter 4: Neck & Spine Massage

The neck and spine are often among the areas of chronic pain. No amount of pain medications can provide effective relief. Pain recurs and is often worse than before.

Tennis Ball Neck Massage

Lie on the floor or sit down with the back to a wall. Trigger points in the neck are better massaged when lying on the floor. The sitting position allows for massage over a wider area, including the shoulders and back.

Place the ball under the neck. Put enough pressure to cause a mild and comfortable ache. Reduce the weight on the ball if the pain becomes uncomfortable or sharp. The pain should gradually decrease or disappear throughout the massage. Stop if the pain worsens during the massage.

Avoid rolling the ball. The pressure from the weight of the head and neck should be enough to relieve the trigger points. Just hold the tennis ball over the aching spots for a few seconds. Hold it until the pain or knot decreases. If the pain becomes uncomfortable, roll the ball a little towards the side. If no improvement is felt in 30-

60 seconds, try another spot. Pain may come from several trigger points so move on to get to other spots.

Spots to Concentrate On

Common trigger points to concentrate on during the massage include the following:

- Upper neck area located just below the skull. When massaging this area, it may be necessary to hold the ball in place with a cupped hand. Lay the head back on a pillow with the hand and the ball underneath. Relax and just let the ball release the constriction from the trigger points.

- Another site is a little above the blades of the shoulder, 4 to 5 inches from the neck's base or from the spine.

- The back of the shoulder is also a possible trigger point. To locate the point, hold the arm against the side of the body. Measure two to three inches above the point where the crease on the armpits stops. Place the ball here and apply a bit of pressure.

- The lateral side of the shoulder over the deltoid muscle area is also one common trigger point. Measure 1-2 inches from the tops of the shoulder and apply pressure using the tennis ball.

- Locate the bump at the base of the neck. Move 2 inches lower and then 1 inch off to either side of the bones of the spine. Apply pressure on these areas.

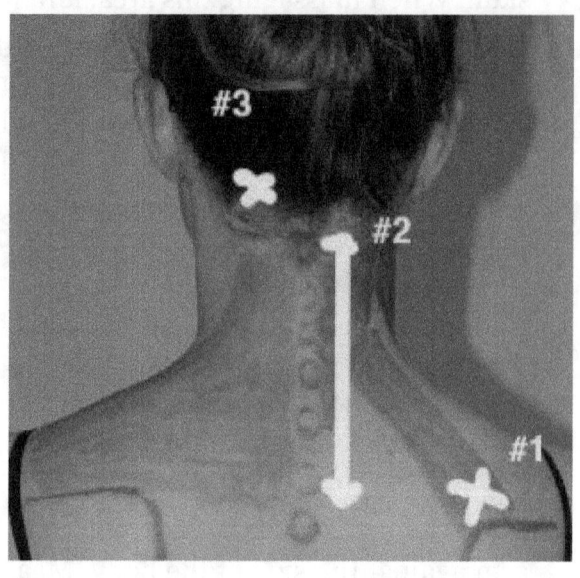

Source: http://www.athletestreatingathletes.com/self-muscle-massage/self-muscle-massage-pt-12-the-neck/

Spinal Tennis Ball Massage

Muscles around the spine are important to maintain an erect posture. These muscles also maintain the normal curvature of the spine.

The muscles are arranged parallel to the bones of the spine. They are also connected and work with the oblique muscles at the sides of the abdomen. When these paraspinal muscles develop trigger points and become tight, back pain happens. It may even go up and contribute to neck pain and headaches. Tennis ball massage therapy can help in relieving the tensions.

To apply the pressure, the tennis ball is placed between a hard surface (floor, wall or firm bed) and the back. Roll the ball until a tender spot is found. Press on it and keep the pressure until it is strong enough to create a good, mild and comfortable ache.

Tennis Ball Massage with the Wall

This is easy and very effective in relieving trigger points along the spine. This is also known as the standing compression method. The amount of compression or pressure is easily controlled by just leaning towards or away from the wall. Stand with the back against a wall.   Place a tennis ball inside a knee-length sock. Hang this across the back, over the shoulders. Lean back against the ball. Lower the ball slowly down the back, along the spine. With each painful spot, stop and lean back. Then move along further downwards.

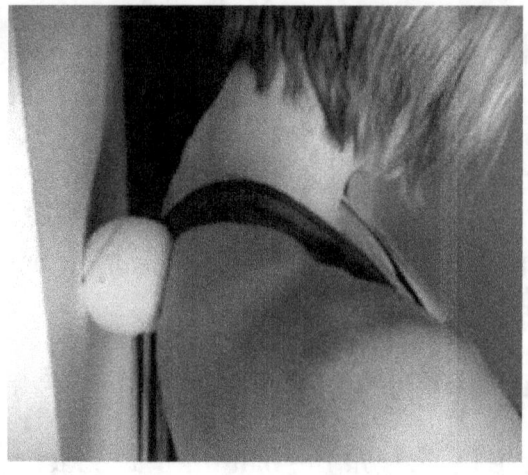

Source: http://wonderwoman.intoday.in/story/soothe-overworked-muscles-with-a-tennis-ball/1/106466.html

Lying Massage

Doing the trigger point tennis ball massage is also effective when done lying down. This position gives a deeper compression than the standing method. Gravity adds to the pressure by pulling much of the body weight down unto the ball. However, control over the amount of applied pressure is less than when standing up.

To perform this method, lie flat with the back on the floor, the knees bent and the feet flat on the floor. Place the tennis ball underneath the lower back. Walk the feet forwards so that the body rolls over the ball. This will bring the ball upwards towards the neck. Rest the hands on the floor, on either side of the body, for balance and support during the exercise.

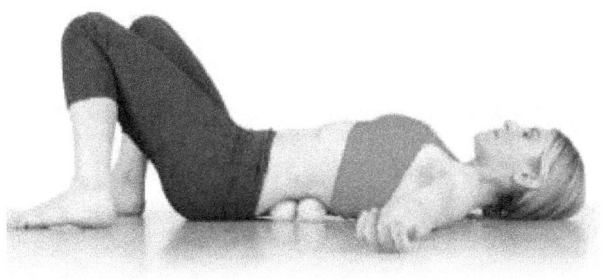

Source: http://www.prevention.com/fitness/fitness-tips/natural-pain-relief-tennis-ball

Massage while Driving

Tennis ball massage over trigger points along the spine can also be performed even while driving. Long drives can cause painful muscle contractions along the back from prolonged sitting. Relieve the tension by performing this massage.

Place the tennis ball between the back and the seat. If driving, have a passenger roll the ball until trigger points are located. Lean back on the ball to put more pressure. If no one is around to assist, pull over the side of the road or a parking lot to do this massage.

Chapter 5: Massage for the Back

Back pains affect everyone. Medications do not work for long and the pain keeps building up. The trapezius muscle over the upper back and the back of the neck are prone to develop trigger points that cause back pains.

Symptoms

Referred pain from these trigger points vary, depending on what portion of the trapezius muscle is affected. There are 3 major divisions of this muscle: the upper, the middle and the lower portions.

Symptoms related to trigger points in the upper trapezius

- Tension headaches, often felt over the temples

- Pain felt behind the eyes

- Pain felt over the jaw and face

- Severe pain over the neck

- Vertigo or dizziness

- Stiffness in the neck

- Inability to tolerate much weight on the shoulders

- Restrictions in the range of motion

Symptoms related to trigger points in the middle trapezius

- Pain over the middle portion of the back

- Headaches felt at the skull's base

- Aching pain felt over the top portion of the shoulders, located in the vicinity of the shoulder joint

- Burning pain superficial in nature felt close to the area of the spine

Symptoms related to trigger points in the lower trapezius

- Pain over the neck, region of the upper shoulders and/or the middle part of the back

- Headaches over the skull's base

- Referred pain over the back part of the shoulder blades radiating down the inner length of the arm and towards the ring finger and the little finger

- Diffuse muscle tenderness and deep aching pain over the top portions of the shoulder

Causes and Precipitating Factors

There are conditions that may force the trapezius muscles to compensate, making it more prone to develop trigger points. These include:

- Uneven lengths of the legs, one is longer than the others

- Uneven measurements of the hemipelvis, one side is smaller than the other

- Upper arms are short, which may lead to the need to lean on one side when using armrests

- Weight from large breasts

- Pectoralis major muscle is tight

There are also some activities that may lead to the development of trigger points, such as:

- Recurrent tensing of the shoulders

- Fatigue

- Cradling the phone between the shoulder and the ear

- Sitting for long periods on chairs with armrests that are too high or those that have no armrests

- Typing on a keyboard placed too high

- Resting sewing materials without any adequate arm support

- Jogging

- Playing violin

- Sleeping while the head is rotated towards the side

- Engaging in activities that require sudden movements in one side only

- Sitting in a slumped position, or in a chair without any firm support for the back

- Prolonged or long term Kayaking, bike-riding or backpacking

- Hiking up one shoulder when carrying something

- Experiencing a whiplash, such as during a car accident or falling on one's head

- Posture with the head leaning forward

- Using a long walking cane

- Keeping the head turned to one side for long period, such as when having a conversation

Clothing can also contribute to the development of trigger points in the trapezius muscles, such as the following:

- Frequent wearing of heavy coats that don't fit well

- Wearing ill-fitting bras, which are too tight over the torso or shoulder straps

- Carrying daypacks, purses or handbags that are too heavy

Some employments are also more prone for this type of problem because their work requires bending over for long periods. This includes work that requires the use computers, dentists and hygienists, draftsmen, secretaries and architects.

How to Apply Pressure

Proper application of pressure using a tennis ball is very important in releasing the trigger points. Follow these simple steps:

- Lie with the back flat on the floor or on a firm bed. Bend the knees.

- Place the tennis ball between the shoulder and the floor (or bed). Position it an inch from the spine. Hold it in place for 8-60 seconds. Roll the ball a little distance downwards and hold it in place. Repeat this until the ball reaches the lower edge of the rib cage. Repeat on the other side of the spine. Avoid placing pressure directly on the spine.

Other methods can be used to place pressure on specific portions of the trapezius muscle. These include the following steps:

For Pain in the Upper Back

Stand with the back leaning against the wall. Position the tennis ball halfway between the spine and the shoulder blades. Lean back on the ball and hold the position for a few seconds. Then move slowly on the ball, up and down, back and forth, rolling it around the area. Make sure to keep the ball within a small area while moving it around. Avoid rolling the ball directly over the spine. Repeat the process on the other side of the back.

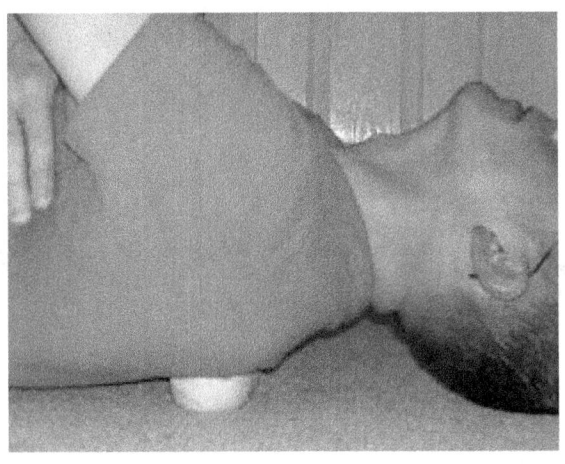

For Pain in the Lower Back

Lie flat on the back (either on the floor or firm bed). Stretch the legs out in front. Position the tennis ball on the spot where the spine and the pelvis meet, about one inch to the side. Again, do not put the ball directly over the spine. Roll the ball horizontally, bringing it towards the hips. Roll it back again. Do this a few more times. Next, roll the tennis ball vertically. Bring the ball from the pelvis up towards the rib cage. Bring the ball back down again. Repeat a few more times.

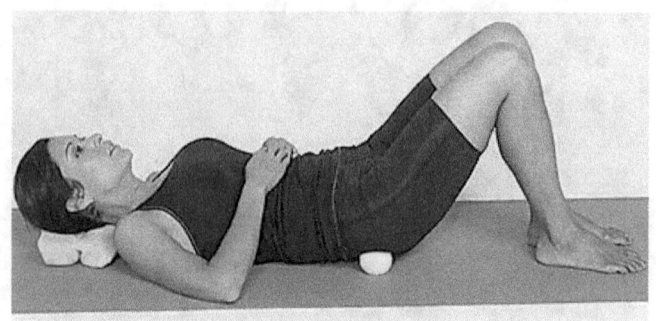

Conclusion

Again, thank you for purchasing this book.

I hope this book was able to help you in relieving those persistent pains over the neck, back and hips. These steps are simple enough to do alone; and can also be performed in the comfort of the home before starting the day or at the end of a long day at work. This can also be done any time in the office or school.

The next thing you should do is to start using the trigger point massage method and ease those pains away. Best of all, tell others about this book. Let them know the wonders that a simple tennis ball can do.

Bonus Content

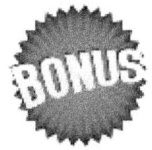

As a token of our appreciation Grand Reveur Publications would like to give you access to our exclusive bonus content (including free eBooks!).

You will be able to acquire exclusive pre-release access to our latest eBooks as well as Free Grand Reveur eBooks during promotional periods.

To simply receive this bonus content please visit the following web site:

https://ignorelimits.leadpages.net/grandreveur publications/

As this is a limited time offer it would be a shame to miss out, I recommend grabbing these bonuses as soon as possible.